Belly Fat Cure

~

10 Foods That Help Burn off Stomach Fat and Bonus Fat Melting Recipes.

Sonja Morgan

Sonja Morgan

Table of Content

Introduction

I want to thank you and congratulate you for purchasing the book,

"Belly Fat Cure: 10 Foods to Help Burn off Stomach Fat and Bonus Fat Melting Recipes."

Belly fat. Hearing it for the first time makes you feel like you are cursed. Cursed in such a way that you feel nothing good is ever going to happen to you again. This is just like each day in which your routine starts with an alarm and you wake up with crazy and frizzy hair. Having belly fat does nothing but degrade your self-image.

As you move on with your day after a quick breakfast and shower, you now think that everything will work out – until you put on your favorite shirt, and it no longer fits. Everything goes downhill from here. You think about things that seem to be working against you, and it feels like the universe is conspiring to make you look and feel bad. A resounding question echoes inside your head, *"Why is this happening to me?"*

By rewinding what happened during the day, you find yourself looking in front of the mirror. Everything seems to be workable – the bad hair, some pimple breakouts, and the laugh lines that you don't regret at all. You even check your smile and how your pearly whites complement your face. Suddenly, your eyes zero into the unsightly view of your bulging midsection.

"Where did that come from?"

"That wasn't even there last week."

Then the reality that you already have belly fat starts to sink in. The situation of having belly fat is something that cannot be denied for obvious reasons. Nowadays, belly fat is considered a norm, but being part of the normal society doesn't mean you shouldn't do anything about it. Belly fat signifies physical and emotional stress; that is why it is important to take heed and act fast.

This is why I wrote this book. I want to help you achieve a better self-image and greater confidence by sharing with you how you can rid yourself of belly fat by knowing which foods to eat and what meals to prepare.

In this book, I will guide you through an exciting journey towards achieving a healthier body and a happier state of mind.

Thanks again for purchasing this book. I hope it is helpful to you!

Copyright © 2015 - Sonja Morgan

Disclaimer

Any received slight of any individual or organization is purely unintentional.

CHAPTER 1

The Curse Of The Belly Fat

Some people might say that acting fast to remove belly fat is easier said than done, and this actually holds a grain of truth in it. In today's ever-changing world and fast-paced lifestyle, we tend to be overwhelmed by our daily routines, so much so that we no longer pay *that much* attention to what we eat. The smell of bacon being fried to a crisp, the view of a Big Mac with some fries, and the indulgent evenings of watching your favorite TV series over a pint of ice cream are all too tempting to resist. Life is about the best things, which may include food, but if you are not careful, you might find yourself overindulging. There are a lot of available routines or disciplines that would allow you to eat whatever you want but with smaller portions, but this approach is not very effective because of the significant amount of self-control and discipline required. Seriously, who wants to deprive themselves of the goodness of fried food and chocolate? No one.

However, overindulgence has certain consequences. Those extra fries and chips that you thought won't matter will accumulate and converge in one of your body parts that has a strong propensity for storing fat – the midsection. The sad thing is that the belly becomes an unsightly body feature that suddenly appears right before you know it. It just says, "Hello World" one morning.

What does your belly do to you?

It is quite normal to have some fat around the abdominal area. However, if the fat this goes beyond what can be considered normal and starts occupying more space, a belly forms.

The abdominal area is one of the most prominent parts of the body where excess fat is stored, especially in men. The midsection, along with the thighs, buttocks, and chest, serve as the major storage areas of fat in the human body. The belly, which is also called pot belly or beer belly, is clinically termed as central obesity. This occurs when an excess buildup of abdominal fat occurs around the abdominal area or stomach. Such excessive buildup may likely pose a negative effect on your health. Excessive fat causes major body organs to go haywire, thus resulting in numerous medical conditions that will definitely affect your quality of life and will have huge implications in how well you can enjoy your future as you age. Research shows that a strong correlation exists between central obesity and cardiovascular disease. Having a bulging belly is also related to other health complications, such as Alzheimer's disease, diabetes, and other metabolic diseases.

These repositories do more than just cause you to gain unwanted pounds. Physically, the belly gives you a pudgy look, which you feel you can live with, but psychologically, you tend to lose your precious self-esteem as you begin to believe that you are inferior to *others* — those who look as if they can appear on the airbrushed pages of a magazine. And don't get me started on the physiological aspect.

Now that's kind of scary, isn't it?

A scientific explanation behind belly fat build up and what you can do to address this problem will be discussed in the next chapter, so you may want to put that French fry down and listen up.

CHAPTER 2

The Science Of Fatness

Scientists formally label belly fat as visceral fat. Now you may ask why it is important to learn about visceral fat and specifically target it as you start your adventure toward burning belly fat. The answer lies in the fact that in terms of negatives effects that can be prevented, if we take care of the bulge as early as possible, visceral fat ranks way up there with head trauma in the leadings causes of death over the past five years. The values are indeed that high. The only difference that separates head trauma and visceral fat is that the former will have instantaneous effects that may threaten your life and your chances of survival. Meanwhile, the effects of visceral fat are not immediately evident, but they pose a serious threat to your well-being, and yes, even to your chances of survival because of the dearth of diseases associated with it.

Belly fat is like the tip of an iceberg that hides a large health problem, or multiple problems in most cases. These health problems can either be cardiovascular or metabolic.

Where does all the fat come from?

There are numerous factors that can contribute to the unwanted accumulation of fat and eventually lead to obesity. An unhealthy diet, one of the usual suspects, along with lack of activity or a sedentary lifestyle, causes the body to store the excess calories in the form of fat. This leads to a gradual increase in your total body mass. One of the most overlooked factors, although considered uncommon, is the lack of sleep. Fewer hours of sleep can trigger hormonal changes, which may increase your appetite. That increase in appetite can work hand-in-hand with the sedentary lifestyle, thus causing you to gain weight and form a fat belly.

There are several sad realities behind belly fat. The brain is primed to crave foods that are high in carbohydrate and caloric content. While it is true that carbohydrates contain very important compounds that aid the body in producing the energy needed for day-to-day activities, the lifestyle that you have defeats this purpose most of the time. When the supply is overwhelming when compared to the activity being done, the body does not burn all the calories that you consume. This leads to fat accumulation, and the end consequence is weight gain.

Women are also placed in a greater disadvantage, especially ladies who have already been pregnant. Given that storing essential minerals and nutrition is an internal body process, weight gain becomes a part of pregnancy to sustain fetal development. As the mother delivers the child, the accumulated fat doesn't go out with the baby. Unfortunately, it stays in the mother's body, and due to hormonal changes, it becomes a very tough challenge to remove the excess fat.

Medications are among the greatest contributions of science and continuous research. While these medications have been formulated to treat illnesses or symptoms effectively, their adverse effects are sometimes not completely explored. Some medications are tied to several side effects that may look simple and manageable at first, but these side effects can actually become a burden in the long run. Some steroids and anti-seizure medications, as well as medications for depression and diabetes, have weight gain and sleeplessness as some of their side effects. Weight gain is an outright problem that can increase the chances of belly formation, whereas sleeplessness is a slower version of this concern. You may say that this may seem unfair, but some side effects are simply unavoidable and serve as a compromise to achieving a greater good, which is specifically targeting the more serious illness.

Research confirms that there is a close relationship between belly fat formation and lipid hypothyroidism, metabolism, obesity, and thermogenesis. This cluster of conditions is difficult to address because individuals with these conditions are in a position that predispose them to being obese.

The next chapter will let you in on some truths about being overweight and will present how you can go from fat to flat. By identifying the pre-existing factors that cause your belly fat, you can take action and address the problem using the available interventions to gain back a healthy you.

CHAPTER 3

The Truth About Being Overweight

Lack of physical activity is considered as one of the most common misconceptions about being overweight. Individuals who are overweight are pigeonholed as those who stay long hours watching their favorite TV shows or long movie marathons that evolve to become a daily habit. Simply put, overweight people are perceived to be plain lazy without any further explanation. However, the truth is that are several factors that are connected with being overweight. Food hoarding, increased appetite due to a lack of self-control, and other behaviors exhibited and seen on TV are usually exaggerated.

The sad truth is that your genes are also responsible for your belly. Those chocolate slices or overindulgent cakes and pizza are not the only culprits. Your genes can also be responsible for your ordeal. These "fat genes" place you in a genetic predisposition that causes you to have an increased chance of gaining weight. You might think that this could be the end of the road for you because it is all in your DNA, but not all hope is lost. You are only placed at an increased risk and a disadvantageous position. Nevertheless, this is something that you should not worry about. Even if your genes are the culprit and give you a disadvantage, you can still gain total control.

We live in a very fast-paced world, where time is extremely precious. With the list of recommended diet and exercise routines that I will provide, you can and you will win this war against fat. You just need to start with a positive mindset. Keep your eyes on the prize, and focus on becoming a leaner, healthier you.

From Flab to Fab

One of the biggest clichés in the history of humanity is that overweight people are always busy — busy eating, that is. Upsizing your soda, having an extra burger patty, and automatically nodding when asked if "you would like to have fries with that," as well as eat-all-you-can-until-you-pass-out offers are indulgences that contribute to belly fat. Overindulgence is a slow but sure process by which you fill your body with bad cholesterol and overexert your organs, which need to process the food that you eat and cause hormonal and digestive imbalance.

With medical research becoming increasingly advanced and the continuous improvement in medical technology being on your side to combat your problem of having belly fat, what was previously known to be something hopeless has become something that can be addressed. A recent study has been conducted to review the hormone leptin, which is responsible for the feeling of satiation or fullness. Lowering the levels of this hormone in the body has been proven to trigger a feeling that signals the brain that you already ate enough and that your cravings are already satisfied without requiring additional food consumption. Satiation inhibits humans from eating more than what makes them feel full. This reduces the chances of storing unused calories that will be converted into fat.

This all sounds very promising, right? Having the sense of security that everything can be fixed with the help of medical intervention, personal determination, and psychological outlook can go a long way and ultimately help you in combating a fat belly.

As we progress to the succeeding chapters, you will gain knowledge of what should be done to burn belly fat in the most effective and convenient way. When we say convenient, it doesn't mean that you will be completely relying on the given options. It will be a personal battle between you and that round prominence in your midsection, and in every battle, you should come in prepared and ready to win.

The Great Intervention

I have provided some of the important facts about having belly fat, and you now know that its existence is deeply rooted in numerous factors that may or may not affect you. Now that you've been properly oriented about the fact that belly fat, or being overweight for that matter, is not a hopeless case, we can now move on to more serious details.

Today, there are countless advertisements about pills, exercise routines, diets, and some miracle tonics, some of which you may have already tried but with no results. This lack of results may have left you wondering why. Could it be due to a missed dose or a wrong preparation, or is it just one of those false advertisements designed to rake in large sums of money from individuals who are desperately looking for a solution?

I will not be providing you with another program that is doomed to fail. This guide will be filled with food choices that have been revered by nutritionists and fitness experts to be effective in helping even those individuals who are dealing with visceral fat with varying levels of severity. In any kind of procedure aimed at modifying one's lifestyle to achieve results that will improve health and overall well-being, there are two keys to successfully finishing the program and achieving results — commitment and a personal decision to complete it and not just try it.

According to most researchers and fitness experts, some individuals who are overweight or obese actually attempt to try to lose weight. However, they don't try as hard as they should. Motivation and personal goals are some of the things that might serve as the best ingredients to make any program work. Even if you have the best fat-melting pill or the greatest exercise routine man has ever made, if you do not take any initiative, nothing will ever work for you. If you feel as if don't have the personal goal or motivation, you should work on finding such motivation fast. This will be your greatest hurdle, and you have to run past that. If you succeed, you will have one of the best life-changing experiences that you can ever have.

The succeeding details about the actions that you can try to burn belly fat will serve as your guide toward achieving what brings you here – to reduce and even totally eliminate belly fat and keep it that way for a very long time. Again, the effectiveness of any of these will still depend on you and how far your will can take you on this battle against the bulge.

CHAPTER 4

Ingredients That Target Belly Fat

Contrary to the popular belief that eating common household food items will increase the chances of gaining weight and creating a fat belly, there are actually a lot of selections that can help you customize your food choices without compromising taste and variety. You just need to be well aware of which food items are better than others. In this way, your body will be able to benefit from the effect of the ingredients that you are consuming to gain the maximum advantage against fat accumulation.

Oils and Healthy Fats

While the phrase "fight fire with fire" can be a little over the top, the truth is that you can actually fight the formation of a fat belly by getting a sufficient supply of oils and healthy fats. Some may be too skeptic to consider that fats themselves are included in the intervention to fight fats. In reality, there are several healthy oils and fat selections that can actually help you address your hunger. Olive oils, virgin coconut oils, as well as foods such as cashews and sardines, can actually do the trick and make you feel full, such that you feel no urge to eat more. This inhibits the need to take appetite suppressant medications that carry unwanted adverse effects with them. These oils and healthy fats can trick the brain into believing that what has been consumed is already enough. This is quite evident when you eat about half a cup full of nuts and you feel stuffed.

Omega 3 Fatty Acids

Since the discovery and proper utilization of Omega 3, researchers and nutritionists have been working collaboratively to determine the primary sources of this fatty acid. Omega 3 fatty acids assist in promoting muscle repair and reducing inflammation. Aside from vegetables and spices, you have a wide range of food choices that have an anti-inflammatory effect. Anchovies, herring, and chia seeds, among others, contain Omega 3 fatty acids that aid in muscle repair and reduce inflammation.

Consuming foods rich in this nutrient can serve as a holistic management for individuals who are trying the gym for the first time or those who are physically challenged and cannot engage in more strenuous routines.

Oats and Beans

Oats and beans have been previously listed as "bad" because they are heavily filled with carbohydrates. Nowadays, this reputation is slowly shifting toward gluten which is a protein composite found in wheat. Gluten can be one of the underground causes of cardiovascular diseases and Alzheimer's disease. This is why it is strongly advised that you maintain a gluten-free diet as much as possible. Beans, as well as lentils, oats, and quinoa, contain two important nutrients that fight cortisol, a stress hormone that stimulates the storage of fat. These ingredients basically intercept the process of fat storage, enabling your body to excrete the excess fat instead of storing it. Also, oats and beans aid in reducing insulin production, elevated levels of which encourage fat to pile up and form in the belly.

Lean Meat

Lean meat can help promote muscle building and repair. This food also shuts down the genes that are responsible for storing excess fat. Lean meat satisfies the protein requirement of the body without the excess bulk.

Green Leafy Vegetables

The regular consumption of green leafy vegetables is proven to reduce the inflammation of tissues and muscles. This is the main reason why gym enthusiasts incorporate healthy greens into their meal plan. Now, for individuals who have no gross pain or inflammation, green leafy vegetables are rich in essential nutrients that keep your RDA on point.

Eggs

Eggs are considered to be among the most amazing foods available. Abundantly filled with essential nutrients that are good for you, eggs are capable of nullifying visceral fat genes. This means that the regular consumption of eggs will actually help you trim down your visceral fat. The earlier claim that eggs are the culprits behind the accumulation of excess cholesterol and fat in the body has been debunked, and eggs have been proven to actually help you.

Red or Reddish Fruits and Vegetables

Considered as the color that stimulates appetite and initiation of meals, red-colored fruits and vegetables not only give color to bland-looking dishes and smoothies, but also give a boost in nutritional value and your body's fat-busting capability. There are a lot of red-colored ingredients available, from bell peppers, to tomatoes, to strawberries, and even grapefruit.

Spices

Spices not only add taste and flavor to our meals, but also provide inflammation-reducing benefits. Black pepper, turmeric, and even cinnamon, among other common spices, have this effect. In addition, spices actually improve blood circulation and raise body temperature. This allows the proper utilization of nutrients and promotes digestive process, as the stomach works better with warmer temperatures, which stimulate gastric juice production. While peppery foods are believed to stimulate the appetite by setting off the flow of saliva and gastric juices, a controlled amount of spices can improve indigestion, as well as decrease fat absorption.

Yogurt

Back in the early nineties, yogurt has been considered a healthier snack option than ice cream and brownies and whatever else that gives you a sugar rush. It contains probiotics that aid digestion and is generally free from artificial ingredients. However, unwanted effects now overshadow these two benefits. Most of the yogurts available in the market are sweetened, even those labeled as unsweetened. For this reason, we strongly discourage the consumption of more than three servings of yogurt a week. This is also the reason why yogurt did not make it into our list of food options.

Chocolate

As long as it is consumed in moderation and as long as you consume the dark variety, chocolate is actually good for you. Gut bacteria can actually break down chocolate into anti-inflammatory compounds that are beneficial to heart health, thanks to flavonoids that are richly contained by darker chocolate varieties. Remember the fad idea of eating chocolate cake for breakfast? Technically, it does work, but only when properly timed.

Another feature that chocolates have is that they contain endorphins. Endorphins are natural hormones produced by the brain that generate feelings of pleasure and promote a sense of well-being. Chocolate may also make a person feel better. When a person who is dealing with belly fat feels bad about his or her physical appearance, endorphins can actually help improve mood and behavior. This makes the overall belly fat management easier to deal with and overcome.

Fiber Power

The marvel of dietary fiber mainly works in two ways. First, it cleanses the digestive system and enhances your body's ability to produce low-density lipoproteins, or LDLs, which have the capability of eliminating bad cholesterol from your blood and improving the blood flow in the entire body by reducing the potential of accumulating plaque in the blood vessels. Second, it improves digestion and cleanses the colon from accumulated cholesterol and toxin buildup that may have been caused by excessive drinking, eating, or a slow digestive process.

Healthcare providers have always highlighted that people with larger waists die earlier than those with flatter bellies, regardless of whether they are within the normal weight range. The fat that envelopes the midsection not only gives an impression that the individual is lazy, but also serves as a precursor of multiple health problems that may rise in the long run. The fat that is stored in the abdominal area increases the risk for cardiovascular disease, stroke, and even diabetes.

CHAPTER 5

Tips In Modifying Your Routine And Achieving Great Results

Several factors can be considered to make any belly fat-melting approach work. Some of these factors can be difficult for starters, but think of the possibilities you can reach and the main reason why you started. It is important to stay focused, remain motivated, and establish self-discipline. These are some of the things that no fitness instructor, dietitian, or instruction manual can force you to do – it should come from within.

Reduce, if not Completely Stop, your Saturated Fat Intake

The first step is usually the hardest. Sure, the sight of a burger platter with fries and soda can make your mouth water. How about breakfast with crisp bacon? These are great, and they are undeniably delicious. If this has been your lifestyle for the longest time, I strongly suggest that you modify it and reduce your intake if complete cessation is not possible at the moment. By cutting down your consumption of saturated fats, you also cut the risks for cardiovascular diseases and other hormonal and metabolic diseases. If you're on a daily bacon or fried chicken routine, try to wean yourself gradually toward a thrice-weekly consumption. Then, if you think you can go further, go once weekly.

The Magic of a Quick Morning Walk

A good morning walk can actually give you more benefits aside from receiving your daily dose of Vitamin D. Morning walks jumpstart the body into functioning properly, which directly involves the heart, muscular system, and the digestive system. It also allows the bones to mobilize after a good night's sleep. Also, walking greatly improves circulation, and the integumentary system is also triggered to function well by controlling the body temperature through sweating. There has been a constant increase in the number of studies that support the benefits of having a morning walk on a daily basis as a holistic method for staying healthy.

Skip the Pills

Vitamins are everywhere nowadays. Clinical studies indicate that they work, but only for those with confirmed vitamin or nutrient deficiency. However, it may not be the same case for individuals who don't have these deficiency problems. Recent studies are starting to provide concrete evidence that taking vitamins is a waste of money. Your body has the capability to extract the vitamins and minerals it needs, given that your digestive system has a far more effective way of collecting nutrients than what synthetic vitamins claim. Vitamins also overload your system, which may lead to hypervitaminosis. This condition can actually become harmful instead of being helpful to your body.

Careful with the Canned

Canned foods are usually filled with preservatives to prolong freshness, and you don't want that stuff in your body. Always check the label to determine the type of preservative, if any, that is present, and always look for better food choices. Another concern is that preserved foods that have been on the shelf for extended periods can be a portal for bacterial growth, especially when the cans become dented or disfigured. Always check the physical appearance of the can. If it is misshapen or rusty, skip it.

Take Your Medication only when Needed

Antibiotics are meant to treat infection. They are generally effective, but they should only be taken when necessary. Antibiotics, although meant to treat bacterial diseases, can also harm the good bacteria inside your digestive system. Please refrain from self-medicating, because it can lead to untoward reactions, especially when the diagnosis is not definite and you are basing your medical management only on previous experiences. When you think you are having an illness or an infection, it would be best to consult your doctor.

CHAPTER 6

The Rewards Of Burning Belly Fat

What is a game plan without the rewards that await you, right? Here are just some of the rewards of successfully burning belly fat. This is a compilation of rewards that can be felt the moment you start seeing results of shrinking belly fat.

You'll lose weight

We will start with the greatest reward of burning belly fat. This should be where your objectives lead. The best benefit of following these recommendations actually goes deeper than the physical feeling of being lighter and looking better. Losing weight will actually make you feel good about yourself and will enable you to gain back the confidence that may have lost when you started to pile on the pounds. Losing weight and burning the belly fat will build better things – your confidence and your health.

Get More from the Food You Eat

Remember that you should not deprive yourself of food choices. What you can do is to be smart with your selection. Food itself is not bad for you. Eating right will let your body collect and absorb the nutrients that it needs to stay healthy and fight illness.

Significant Decrease in Risk of Chronic Disease

Just hearing the words *chronic disease* is enough to scare people. The good news is that losing weight and having a flatter belly will actually reduce your risk of developing any chronic disease, even as you age.

Less Chances to Catch a Cold

This is actually a bonus that may come in handy. Due to the rapid changes in the weather, your body is bound to catch the common cold. The association lies in the fact that burning belly fat leads to a healthier you – which means a healthier immune system as well.

Your body will start manufacturing fatty acids that shut down genes that make you fat

Remember what I said about fat genes being a culprit? While it is true that genes cannot be changed, they can actually be reprogrammed, such that they no longer work to increase fat storage. If this will be your body's regular mechanism, you will be able to utilize the best things by maximizing the nutrition that you are currently receiving. Your body has the ability to manufacture fatty acids. However, this is either an underpowered ability or is overpowered by bad food choices in the past.

Better Overall Well-Being

Nothing feels better than being comfortable with yourself, both inside and out. With the absence of a distracting fat belly, you feel better and become healthier.

CHAPTER 7

Key Habits Of Successful Losers

Yes, you read that right. These are the key habits of successful losers. If you are on a struggle because these things are becoming such a hurdle in your endeavor of burning belly fat, then go on a detour and change your mindset and game plan.

Never Engage in Crash Diets

Crash diets will literally crush you. Not only will they lead to consequences of calorie and nutritional shortage, they will also result in decreased sensory and logical function. Crash diets should never be tried.

No to Fat-Free

Fat is good, if you are taking the right ones. The main classification of good and bad fats will help you be wise about your food choices. Keep in mind that good fats will inhibit the bad fats and will help you stay healthy.

Do Not Eat and Run

Speed eating will not only cause stomach pains, it can also lead to increased consumption. By eating slowly, you allow your food to be properly chewed or masticated, which means better digestion once it reaches the stomach. It also allows you to enjoy your food more and makes you fuller compared to when you eat in a rush.

Plan Ahead

In conjunction with our do not eat and run policy, it is wise to plan ahead. Planning involves your daily activities, your meal choices, and your schedule. You will feel more accomplished and organized with your activities for the day from sun up to sun down.

Do Not Miss on Protein

Many individuals skip on protein and forget that this nutrient is essential for muscle development, toning, and repair. Muscles that are toned can help you burn more calories, and regular protein intake takes care of the injured muscles – even the muscle fibers that you cannot see.

Stay Active

Staying active does not require you to become a gym rat or a hardcore diet-driven monster. When I say stay active, what I mean is that you should keep yourself mobile. Try physical activities such as walking to a nearby convenience store instead of driving to it or walking the dog by yourself instead of hiring a dog-sitter. You can burn calories in the process and help your body stay fit. When the body is used to being idle and sedentary, fat deposits just stay there. When you mobilize yourself, you activate your fat reserves and inhibit the possibility of fat accumulation.

Turn off the TV

Yes, this is one of the hardest habits to give up. If you can't stop watching, make a compromise and watch only your absolute favorite shows. It is sometimes painful, but it pays off well.

CHAPTER 8

Food Selections

Here are some of the recommended food preparations that are low in carbohydrate content, but equally filling and satisfying. You might be surprised that there are ingredients here that are irked by traditional dieters (Hint: Bacon), but is considered as a wonderful addition to a healthy dish. Bear in mind that these menus can be modified whichever is the closest ingredient that is available.

Hearty Morning Casserole

Ingredients:

- ¼ tsp. of cracked black pepper
- ¾ tsp. of dry mustard
- 1 tsp. of sea salt
- ½ cup of almond milk
- 6 oz. of bacon, chopped
- ½ lb. of bulk breakfast sausage, crumbled
- 16 eggs (large), beaten
- 1 orange bell pepper, seeds removed then diced
- 1 red bell pepper, seeds removed then diced
- 1 lb. of white sweet potatoes, skin removed then shredded
- ½ cup of yellow onion, diced
- Green onions (as garnish)
- ¼ cup of coconut milk (full-fat)
- Ghee, softened

Instructions:

1. Lightly coat the insert of the slow cooker with softened ghee. The coating should be just well enough to cover the entire insert.

2. In a skillet set on medium-high heat, cook the bacon, sausage, and onion for about 10 to 12 minutes. Once the sausage is evenly browned and onion becomes soft, drain the excess fat from the skillet.

3. Add the white sweet potatoes into the slow cooker, and gently press them down.

4. Add the cooked onion, sausage, and bacon into the slow cooker, along with the red and orange bell peppers.

5. In a mixing bowl, whisk together the salt, coconut milk, almond milk, pepper, mustard, and eggs. Pour the mixture into the slow cooker.

6. Cover and cook for 8 hours on a low setting. Then, give it a quick stir, and transfer it onto a serving dish.

Wheat-Free Pancakes

Ingredients:

- 2 tbsp. of olive oil (extra-light)
- 1 tbsp. of ground flaxseed
- 3 cups of almond meal
- ¾ cup of almond milk (unsweetened)
- 3 eggs (large)
- ½ tsp. of baking soda
- ½ tsp. of sea salt

Instructions:

1. In a mixing bowl, combine salt, baking soda, salt, almond meal, and flaxseed.

2. In another bowl, whisk together the almond milk, olive oil, and eggs. Whisk thoroughly.

3. Gradually whisk in the flour mixture into the eggs. If necessary, you can add more almond milk to achieve the right consistency for a pancake batter.

4. Grease a pan lightly, and set it on medium heat. Pour about ¼ cup of batter into the pan, and cook for 3 minutes. Once the edges are cooked and bubbles form, flip and cook the other side for another 3 minutes. Repeat the same process with the remaining batter.

5. Serve with preferred toppings. Fresh or frozen fruits in season are recommended.

Quick Morning Breakfast Bowl

Ingredients:

- 1 pinch of freshly ground pepper
- juice of 1 lemon
- 2 fresh eggs
- ¼ of an avocado, diced
- ½ cup of arugula
- 2oz of wild smoked salmon
- 1 tsp. of ghee

Instructions:

1. Set a non-stick cooking pan in medium heat. Swirl the ghee around the pan. Gradually add the two eggs into the pan, and cook them for about 6 minutes.

2. Meanwhile, assemble the smoked salmon, avocado, and arugula in a clean bowl. Drizzle the fresh lemon juice on everything, and sprinkle with freshly cracked pepper to taste.

3. Once the eggs are cooked, slide them into the bowl.

4. Serve immediately.

Guiltless and Easy Pizza

Ingredients:

- ¼ tsp. of red pepper flakes (crushed)
- Black pepper, freshly ground
- Kosher salt
- 2 cloves of garlic, sliced
- ¼ cup of tomato sauce
- 2 tbsp. of grated parmesan cheese
- 1 ¼ cups of shredded mozzarella cheese (part-skim)
- 1 egg (large), beaten lightly
- 1 cup of grape tomatoes, halved
- 2 ½ cups of cauliflower, grated
- Non-stick spray

Instructions:

1. Switch on the oven and set it to 425°F. Prepare a rimmed baking sheet, and line it with parchment paper.

2. Place the grated cauliflower in a bowl and microwave for about 8 minutes. Once it becomes soft, take it from the microwave and allow it to cool.

3. Once the grated cauliflower has cooled down, mix in the salt, pepper, parmesan cheese, 1 cup of mozzarella cheese, and egg. Once done, pat it into a lightly greased pizza pan to create a 10-inch round pizza crust. Bake for 15 minutes.

4. Once the crust turns golden brown, top it with the tomato sauce, remaining ¼ cup of mozzarella cheese, grape

tomatoes, red pepper flakes, and garlic. Return it into the oven, and bake for 10 minutes.

5. Once done, let it cool slightly before slicing and serving.

Basic Tortilla Soup

Ingredients:

- Avocado slices (for garnish)
- 28oz of fire-roasted tomatoes (diced)
- 2 quarts of chicken stock
- Juice from 2 limes
- 1 cup of fresh cilantro, chopped
- 1 lb. of chicken breast, cooked then diced
- 1 tbsp. of ghee
- 2 fresh jalapeno peppers, diced
- 6 cloves of garlic, peeled then minced
- 1 yellow onion (large), diced

Instructions:

1. In a Dutch oven set on medium heat, add in the ghee.

2. Then, sauté the yellow onion for 6 minutes.

3. Add in the jalapeno peppers and garlic and sauté for 2 minutes.

4. Pour the tomatoes and chicken stock, and bring the liquid to a boil. Cook for about 5 minutes.

5. Stir in the lime juice, cilantro, and cooked chicken. Then, serve with avocado slices on top.

Blueberry Scones

Ingredients:

- 1 1/2 cups almond flour
- 2 1/4 tsp baking powder
- 1 cup blueberries
- 3 eggs, whisked
- 2/3 cup stevia or coconut sugar
- 2 1/4 tsp pure vanilla extract

Instructions:

1. Set the oven to 375 °F. Prepare a baking sheet by lining it with parchment paper.

2. Put the almond flour in a large bowl and create a well in the center. Add the vanilla, beaten eggs, baking powder, and stevia or coconut sugar as alternative. Mix to combine.

3. Fold in the blueberries carefully, gently mixing until well distributed.

4. Spoon about 3 tablespoons of the batter onto the prepared baking sheet to make one scone. Repeat the process until all of the batter is gone.

5. Bake for about 12 to 15 minutes or until the scones are golden brown.

6. Set on a cooling rack for about 12 minutes before serving.

Grilled Sardines

Ingredients:

- 24 medium sized sardines, cleaned, scales, gills and innards removed
- 1 1/2 tsp sea salt
- Freshly ground black pepper
- 12 Tbsp. extra virgin olive oil
- 6 Tbsp. chopped fresh basil, or 6 tsp dried
- 6 Tbsp. chopped fresh mint

Instructions:

1. Preheat the oven to 350 °F.

2. Rinse the sardines thoroughly under cold running water, then season with salt and pepper.

3. Arrange on the oven rack and bake for 10 minutes. Transfer to a platter and top with chopped mint and basil.

4. Drizzle the olive oil on top, then serve immediately.

Steamed Garlic and Thyme Mussel

Ingredients:

- 6 lb. live mussels
- 2 Tbsp. fresh thyme
- 3/4 cup diced onion
- 1/3 cup olive oil
- 3/4 cup white wine
- 3/4 cup butter
- 6 garlic cloves, minced
- 3/4 cup diced tomato
- 1 1/2 cups broth, chicken or seafood
- 3 tbsp. juice from a freshly squeezed lemon
- 2/3 tsp sea salt
- 1/3 tsp freshly grounded black pepper

Instructions:

1. Clean and scrub the mussels very well, then trim off the beards. Place them in a bowl and fill them with cool water until completely submerged. Set aside.

2. Place a heavy bottomed pot over medium flame and combine the butter and olive oil in it. Once the butter has melted, stir in the onions and cook for about 5 minutes, or until translucent. Stir in the garlic and cook for 1 more minute.

3. Stir in the tomato, thyme, lemon juice, broth, and white wine. Season with salt and pepper, then bring to a boil.

4. Drain the mussels, then add to the pot. Cover and cook for 10 minutes. Shake the pot to redistribute the mussels inside

and allow even cooking. Do not open the lid until after 10 minutes.

5. Transfer the mussels to a bowl. Dispose the mussels those that have not opened. Serve at once.

Easy Prawn and Smoked Salmon Salad

Ingredients:

- 4 tsp Dijon mustard
- 4 Tbsp. extra virgin olive oil
- 7 oz. smoked wild salmon, sliced into thin strips
- 6 cups romaine lettuce, rinsed and drained
- 4 tsp white or red wine vinegar
- 4 Tbsp. fresh dill
- 14 oz. king prawns, boiled or roasted, hard parts removed
- 4 cups halved cherry tomatoes
- Freshly ground black pepper

Instructions:

1. Arrange the lettuce in a salad bowl.

2. Toss together the cooked prawns, halved cherry tomatoes, salmon strips and dill, then pile on top of the lettuce. Season with black pepper.

3. In a bowl, whisk together the olive oil, vinegar, and Dijon mustard. Drizzle over the salad and toss to coat evenly.

4. Serve at once.

Stir Fried Broccoli and Beef

Ingredients:

- 2/3 tsp Chinese five spice powder
- 3 Tbsp. sake
- 3 cloves garlic, minced
- 1 1/2 Tbsp. grated fresh ginger
- 6 cups broccoli florets
- 1 1/2 lb. skirt steak, cut into 1 inch strips and halved
- 4 Tbsp. coconut oil
- 1 1/2 cup diced onion
- 3 Tbsp. soy sauce
- 2/3 cup sliced scallions

Instructions:

1. Combine the ginger, garlic, soy sauce, five spice, and sake in a bowl. Toss in the steak strips to coat. Cover and chill for about half an hour to marinate.

2. Place a wok or skillet over medium high flame and heat the coconut oil. Stir fry the onion until translucent, then add the beef and marinade and stir-fry for 5 more minutes.

3. Stir in the scallions and broccoli for 2 minutes, then cover and set heat to medium low. Let simmer for 3 minutes more to tenderize the broccoli.

4. Mix well then serve at once.

Conclusion

Thank you again for purchasing this book! I really do hope you found it helpful.

Health is something that everyone should treasure. You may indulge in the good things in life, such as food and the joy of living, but you should never neglect nor compromise your health. The goal of burning belly fat is not just a war where you will emerge as the victor once the fat has been cleared. Victory becomes you when you have conquered the battle to fitness and emerged as a better and a healthier person.

Finally, if you enjoyed this book, then I'd like to ask you for a favor, would you be kind enough to leave an honest review of this book on Amazon? It'd be greatly appreciated!

Good Luck and All the Best!!